I0560562

LIVING
WITH
CANCER

LESSONS IN COURAGE,
COMFORT AND CONNECTION

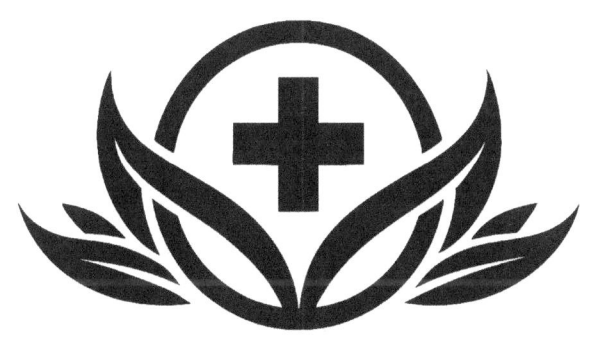

SUSIE WATTS, ARTHUR MOYER

LIVING WITH CANCER: Lessons in Courage, Comfort and Connection

Copyright © 2025 by Susie Watts and Arthur Moyer

All rights reserved.

Formatting provided by Trisha Fuentes

ISBN: 979-8-9890574-3-6 (Paperback)
        979-8-9890574-2-9 (Ebook)

Dedicated to my father

Contents

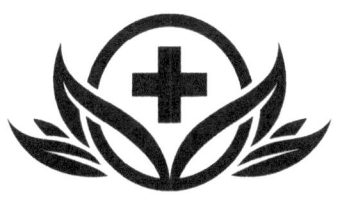

Preface

I remember it well: the phone call, the tears, and the questions I wanted to ask. In that moment, everything changed. My father's voice, usually so strong and reassuring, trembled with a vulnerability I had never heard before. The words "I have cancer" echoed in my mind.

This book is not only my father's journey with cancer, but it also explores the bonds that tie us together. It's about the lessons learned in the face of adversity, the importance of family and friends, and the shared strength that emerges from such an experience. As I write about his journey, I invite you to walk alongside us, to celebrate the victories and witness the struggles that defined this period of time.

A serious cancer diagnosis can be overwhelming, but it can also be a turning point, prompting you to rethink your priorities and explore new paths toward healing and hope. Whether you are a patient, a caregiver, or simply looking to understand the cancer journey better, together we will uncover the strength that lies within you to shape your own course, follow your unique path, and find peace amid uncertainty.

My father wanted this book to provide hope for every reader. He felt it could be a powerful companion when you are facing cancer. It serves as a positive sign in the darkest moments, guiding you on a path through uncertainty and fear. Even during the challenges and setbacks, hope encourages a belief in the possibility of healing and better days ahead.

He wanted to share his experiences in a way that encourages a genuine sense of empathy and understanding. He hoped that his struggles and insights would resonate with your own experiences, allowing you to feel that he understood what you are going through. What he shares here worked for him, and while he cannot promise it will work for everyone, it is worth exploring.

My father had a passion for reading and researching topics that captivated his interest, so he felt compelled to explore what insights were available about coping with cancer. What stood out to him was that the wisdom he uncovered was not groundbreaking; rather, it consisted of timeless principles that have existed throughout human history. The essential takeaway is that each person must discover and internalize these lessons in their own unique way.

As his daughter and coauthor, I encourage you to appreciate each moment, find joy in the small successes, and connect deeply with loved ones. Cultivating hope can help you advocate for your care, explore new treatments, and discover inner strength you never knew existed. This will allow you to create a fulfilling and meaningful life, regardless of the challenges you face.

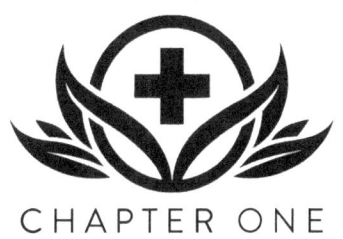

CHAPTER ONE

Beyond the Diagnosis

I was recovering at home after a minor surgery and looking forward to returning to my normal life. At first, everything seemed fine during my recovery. I was resting, healing, and feeling optimistic—until I sensed something was off. I noticed my clothes were fitting a little looser, and the energy I once had for the activities I enjoyed was gone. I felt weak, and I didn't know why.

I decided to reach out to my primary care physician, who suggested I come in for a full check-up. At that moment, it didn't seem important. My wife, Marion, didn't join me because, honestly, it felt like just another routine visit.

But when the test results came back, everything changed dramatically. The inconclusive findings led to more tests, each one feeling like a step deeper into uncertainty. It was during this second round of diagnostics that the dreaded news arrived: advanced lung cancer. The words hit me hard, heavy with meaning.

Life has a way of throwing curveballs when you least expect them. We all know, deep down, we will not last forever, but somehow, we think we are immune to the harsh realities that others face. Hearing that word—cancer—is scary, no matter your age.

I cannot recall the exact phrases the doctor used; what I remember is the weight of his statement: "You have lung cancer, and it's serious." I felt like I was trapped in a movie, watching from a distance as my life fell apart.

I heard him suggest that my wife or kids should contact him for further details, but it all felt like background noise, disconnected from the reality that had just crashed into my world. I was desperately looking for a genuine connection—a lifeline in that moment to pull me from the fear of this ordeal.

Once outside the office, I tried to prepare myself to share the news with my wife. When I got home, I urged her to call the doctor for the specifics that slipped through my understanding at the time. My mind was full of questions, fears soaring out of control. In an instant, hope turned into despair, and I felt lost in a sea of uncertainty.

Because the clues to an illness are sometimes hard to find in the beginning, many of us go through an unavoidable trial-and-error search for the real causes underlying symptoms of cancer.

Looking back on my conversation with the doctor, I remembered my desire for honesty. He had honored that request, explaining the truth in stark detail. While it was difficult to take in, there was a strange comfort in knowing what I was facing. It offered me a sense of control in an otherwise confusing situation.

For many, a clear understanding of their prognosis creates a foundation to make informed decisions. It can encourage conversations with loved ones that might otherwise remain unspoken. Yet the phrase "advanced cancer" can also flood your heart with fear and anxiety, casting a shadow over your future.

Each person struggles with unwelcome news differently; some might prefer to hear unpleasant news gradually, processing it over time, while others may not want to know the full truth at all. I realized how vital it is for healthcare providers to be sensitive to these differences, adjusting their approach to meet the emotional needs of each patient.

A friend of mine once shared that receiving his diagnosis all at once would strip him of hope and motivation. He would much prefer to have the news revealed in stages, not all at one time. This reinforced the importance of a compassionate approach from doctors, creating an environment that helps patients in whatever way suits them best. If confronted with a potentially difficult diagnosis, how would you prefer to hear the results?

As my next appointment with the doctor approached, my stomach churned with a mix of nerves and a flash of hope. A wise friend had suggested bringing someone I trusted along to help take notes, and that turned out to be a great idea. Having someone by my side provided not only emotional support but also a safety net for the key details that I might miss.

Determined to take charge, I put together a detailed list of my symptoms—when they began, their frequency, and how intensely they affected me. I wrote down my concerns and the questions I wanted to ask. This preparation became my way of making sure I would not forget anything important during my time with the doctor. By also opening up about my fears, I felt more supported and understood.

A few days later, even though I was still in a state of disbelief, I made a conscious choice: I did not want to linger on the things I could not control. Instead, I focused on positive lifestyle changes and making self-care practices a part of my daily routine.

By taking these steps, I wanted to shift my thoughts from fear and uncertainty to action and resilience. After all, life is about embracing each moment, even the most difficult ones, and discovering strength in the face of adversity.

I remind myself that while cancer is a part of my journey, it will not define me. My attitude and choices are what I will focus on; these are things within my control. Each day is a gift and an opportunity to find beauty and joy, even during trying times.

PAUSE FOR THOUGHT

Receiving a serious cancer diagnosis can be overwhelming, but keeping a positive attitude can encourage us to face the difficulties ahead with determination and perseverance. Within this challenge lies an opportunity to develop strength, welcome support, and find moments of enjoyment and connection that can guide us through the days ahead. In the end, it is our outlook and relationships that will help us to move forward.

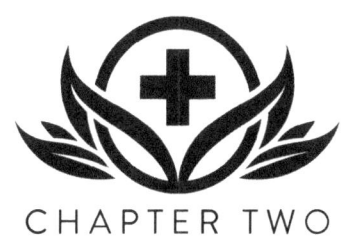

CHAPTER TWO

Mixed Emotions

A week after my diagnosis, I started to feel a strange numbness settling in. It was a disconcerting feeling, as if my body was trying to tell me something I couldn't yet understand. However, during this turmoil, I found unexpected moments of clarity that helped me confront my fears head-on. Oddly enough, it gave me a fresh perspective. No matter what the doctor said, I discovered a surprising sense of peace about the road ahead.

I often thought about how abrupt life can be—like when someone suffers a fatal heart attack and everything changes in an instant, or when a friend quietly passes away after a perfect day on the golf course. But dealing with cancer felt different altogether.

When my doctor broke the news, it became clear that this was more than just a medical issue; it was a life-altering experience. His words hung in the air, reminding me of how fragile life can be. Hearing the phrase "very serious cancer" brought a wave of despair that was difficult to digest, especially for someone like me who had never faced such harsh realities before.

As the weight of the diagnosis sank in, my mind filled with worry, which began to affect my sleep. Nights became a series of restless thoughts and unpleasant fears. The struggle to find peace during those late-night hours only added to the emotional burden, creating a cycle of fatigue and worry that seemed impossible to escape.

When everything was quiet, my mind would start racing. I would lie in bed, tossing and turning, as my thoughts spiraled into a dark unknown. The silence heightened my fears, creating a battleground of emotions. Questions flooded my mind: What does this mean for my future? How will this affect my loved ones? Do I have the strength to face what lies ahead?

Those still nights painted a picture of a life that felt increasingly out of control. It is no surprise that cancer can disrupt sleep; I was certainly no exception. Sleep had not always come easily for me, but after my diagnosis, it became an even bigger issue. I knew that getting quality rest mattered; without it, my emotional and physical health would suffer.

To improve my sleep, I made a few lifestyle changes. I cut out coffee and other caffeinated drinks in the late afternoon, understanding they disrupted my ability to unwind later. I committed to getting outside every day, even if just for a few minutes, to soak up some sun and fresh air while doing some light stretching.

Later, when I was eating more regularly, my wife adjusted our meals, making lunch our biggest meal so I would not have digestive issues at bedtime. These little changes helped lift my mood and promote better sleep.

Of course, not every night was perfect. I found that brief naps during the day could be helpful, but I avoided late-afternoon naps to keep my nighttime sleep on track. Listening to soft music in bed also became part of my routine. It often helped me relax and drift off more easily. Do any of these sleep suggestions sound like they could be helpful for you?

Feeling that I had done what I could to improve my sleep, I was eager to learn more about my cancer. I wondered if this was the right time to dive into research, but my curiosity got the best of me. The information I uncovered included various treatment options, potential side effects, and survival rates, but the overall message was often discouraging.

When facing cancer, it is natural to look for information to find out about your options so you can understand your condition better and make informed decisions. I knew that while researching could be beneficial, it was critical to approach it carefully and with the guidance of my doctors.

The internet can be a mixed bag—there's valuable information out there, but also a lot of misinformation that can create fear and confusion. Your doctor can help you weigh your options and explain how they could affect your treatment.

I learned I could explore mental health support and complementary therapies to improve my overall well-being. Focusing on these aspects can help tackle not just the physical obstacles of cancer but also the emotional and psychological hurdles that come with it. It is all about finding balance and nurturing yourself through this experience.

While relying on family and friends can be critical during this time, I found that many individuals do not have family nearby to support them through their cancer journey. Thankfully, cancer support groups are available for anyone facing similar challenges. Connecting with others who understand what you are going through can be incredibly comforting and helps lessen feelings of isolation.

In these groups, members often share valuable insights from their own experiences, offering practical advice and encouragement that you might not receive elsewhere. The emotional support provided can be a lifeline, encouraging a sense of community that is essential during such difficult times. By participating in these groups, you not only gain support but also realize you are not alone in your journey, which can bring a sense of hope and resilience.

Recently, while I was talking with a friend, she suggested something I found to be particularly helpful. She emphasized the importance of distraction. She could tell I was preoccupied with my illness and suggested I find other ways to focus my attention.

Engaging in activities that took my mind off my disease was extremely helpful. Distractions can serve as a valuable coping mechanism when dealing with a serious illness, as they can help reduce anxiety, lift your mood, and provide moments of enjoyment.

For me, reading was always something I enjoyed, but I had done little of it since my diagnosis. Knowing that I might find it difficult to concentrate, I sought out light and easy reads that wouldn't require a great deal of thought. I found myself drawn to "feel-good" stories and books, and short detective novels that were fun to read and engaging.

I also discovered that music played a significant role in helping me relax. Listening to my favorite music provided a comforting escape and brightened my mood. Others might enjoy activities like crossword puzzles, card games, or creative outlets such as painting or drawing.

Whatever the distraction may be, it can be a helpful tool in managing the difficulties of your illness.

By concentrating on the present moment, I found that I could shift my attention from what I was losing or fearing to the positive things in my life. I learned that worrying about my situation was not helpful and could rob me of my present peace of mind. With each step forward, I focused on the possibilities ahead rather than the limitations.

PAUSE FOR THOUGHT

Processing a cancer diagnosis requires time and space to experience all our emotions, from fear to hope, as we navigate this unpredictable journey. In these moments of reflection, we can start to find meaning even amid the uncertainty. It is essential to remember that each step forward, no matter how small, can lead to a deeper understanding of ourselves and the strength we have to face the unknown. We must trust in our resilience and the support of those around us as we move into uncharted territory.

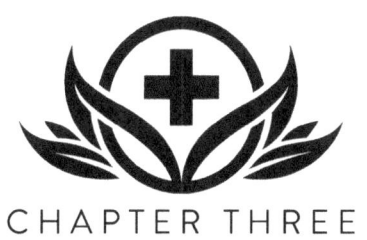

CHAPTER THREE

Strength in the Struggle

Soon after my diagnosis, I was caught off guard by how quickly my wife reached out to family and friends— even those who lived far away. Suddenly, I felt like I was in the spotlight, and honestly, I was not enjoying it. This unsettling attention made it clear to me how serious my illness was. Their encouraging messages reminded me of our deep connections.

While the sudden attention was uncomfortable, it also highlighted the strength of our relationships and the community that surrounds us. Each call, message, and visit reminded me I was not alone on this journey. Maybe this collective support could lighten the burden, changing a frightening experience into something we could share with those who care about us.

As I processed this unsettling diagnosis, I felt a moment of resilience within me. I realized that even though my prognosis was not great, my journey was still mine to navigate. Yes, the unknown can be scary, but it can also be a source of strength, connection, and moments of enjoyment, even during tough times. How do you want to navigate your cancer journey so that you feel in control?

This tug-of-war between despair and hope is something I am learning to manage as I face each day with a blend of courage and a deeper understanding of my circumstances. However, the reality of my situation often weighs heavily on my mind. Like many of us, I had dreams and plans for the future—like visiting our daughter in Denver to spend time with our grandkids.

Now, the thought of making that trip feels almost impossible. Our son lives just two hours away, which used to mean we could see him more often, but even those visits now seem complicated and out of reach.

Closer to home, our social life has shifted significantly. What used to be enjoyable interactions with friends has changed to brief visits from those who understand that I get tired easily. With a prognosis that is not encouraging, it sometimes feels like our future plans are slipping away, but we are finding new ways to cope with this uncertain path.

The quieter moments at home offer us a chance to appreciate the meaningful relationships we have, as those who visit bring care and support into our lives. While our get-togethers may be less frequent, the love and understanding from our friends make each visit even more special.

Talking about my illness with Marion was nearly impossible. The emotions were just too raw. There were times we would sit together but avoid eye contact, as if the weight of unspoken words hovered in the air.

Whenever we tried to have a serious conversation about my diagnosis, tears were never far behind. I later learned that this kind of emotional distance is common, but it was a new and awkward experience for us. It often felt as though we were speaking different languages, struggling to understand one another's feelings. I hope that with time, we can communicate better.

I felt fragile. Mornings were tough, and breakfast—once my favorite meal—now felt like a chore. I simply had no appetite. After forcing myself to glance at the newspaper or watch a brief news clip on TV, I would often go back to bed to rest.

Lunchtime came and went, but I struggled to eat much. While I tried to read the paper, I found it hard to concentrate; I would often stare blankly into space. By the time evening rolled around, I would try to eat whatever I could and then usually go back to bed.

Throughout this time, thoughts of my illness were always there, lurking in the background. The word "cancer" hit hard, and on top of that, my doctor discovered an internal infection, leading to complications from my prescribed medications and leaving me even weaker.

You might notice that your relationships with family and friends can shift after a cancer diagnosis. This transition can be frustrating, as the people in your life may not always know how to respond to your situation.

While many do their best to offer support, their well-intentioned actions or words may sometimes lead to misunderstandings, leaving you feeling isolated and misunderstood. It is important to recognize that this is an emotional experience that adds layers of complexity to your interactions.

You find yourself not only managing your own feelings of fear, anxiety, and sadness but also dealing with the responses and emotions of those around you. This creates a delicate balance between prioritizing your own self-care needs and addressing the emotional needs of your loved ones, which can sometimes feel overwhelming.

Open communication becomes critical, as it helps bridge the gap between your experience and their understanding, creating deeper connections during this difficult time. Amid this emotional turmoil, my illness suddenly turned my wife into my caregiver. This was uncharted territory for both of us. We were fortunate that neither of us had needed long-term care before. I hoped that being a caregiver might bring her some fulfillment, but I also knew it could be distressing.

I encouraged her to read as much as she could about my type of cancer and the treatment options available. Since I wanted to maintain as much independence as possible, I suggested I handle whatever I could on my own; this would help me feel more in control and boost my self-esteem.

Although we had talked little about my diagnosis so far, I shared my hope that we could soon express our feelings and fears more openly. I knew she would experience a range of emotions too, and I wanted her to feel comfortable talking with me instead of bottling everything up.

I also let her know that I would need her help to manage medications and keep track of appointments, as well as provide moral support. I encouraged her to reach out to friends and family for her own emotional encouragement and to remember the importance of continuing a life outside of caregiving.

Taking breaks and allowing herself time to recharge would help both of us during this trying time. What steps can you take to help your spouse feel more comfortable in the role of caregiver?

PAUSE FOR THOUGHT

Moving forward after a cancer diagnosis involves embracing a new chapter of life with courage and determination, focusing on both healing and personal growth. Each day offers a chance to redefine what is possible, celebrate small successes, and connect with loved ones who provide unwavering support. This experience may be challenging, but it also reveals inner strength and perseverance. Ultimately, it teaches us to appreciate the beauty in the journey, no matter how difficult it may be.

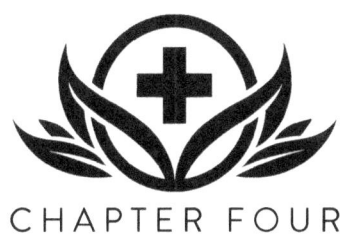

CHAPTER FOUR

The Power Within

Ten days after my initial diagnosis, I had another appointment with my primary care physician. I never thought I would make it. Getting dressed, getting into the car, getting out of the car, and walking to his office felt almost impossible, but I made it. The doctor was late, which only added to my anxiety.

As I asked numerous questions, he answered them truthfully, but they were not always the responses I wanted to hear. Each of his words felt heavy, weighing down the fleeting hope I was desperately trying to hold on to.

I could see the compassion in his eyes, but his straightforwardness made it hard for me to fully grasp the reality of what I was facing. He mentioned chemotherapy as an option but warned me it probably wouldn't be effective for my type of cancer. The doctor provided the name of an oncologist and suggested I call him for specialized treatment.

We scheduled an appointment with the oncologist, and I was eager to begin whatever treatment was necessary, hoping that the path ahead would provide clarity and open doors to healing. The doctor was young but appeared genuinely knowledgeable, which gave me confidence that I was in capable hands.

Our first meeting took place in the examining room. I changed into my boxers for a thorough examination. As he checked me over, we continued our conversation. When it was time to get dressed, I struggled to put my socks back on.

He asked if I had dressed myself, and I replied that I had. He seemed surprised, mentioning that many of his cancer patients needed help. I wondered if I would ever reach a point where I could not dress myself. The thought of such dependence was unsettling, and I certainly did not want to place that burden on my wife. To me, that would feel like giving up entirely. I was not ready to do that!

After the exam, we moved into his office to talk more. I expressed my belief in facing this disease with dignity and courage, highlighting the importance of sharing my feelings. I wanted him to understand that while I was not afraid of the future, I had concerns about the difficulties ahead. "I mean the pain," I said.

To my relief, he assured me that significant pain was not something most patients experienced, and effective pain management options were available for those who needed them. I mentioned that when the time came for medication, I would be open to it and that I had no fears about being labeled a "substance abuser." This conversation not only provided clarity but also offered a sense of hope, knowing that there are ways to navigate this journey with comfort and support.

We also briefly discussed chemotherapy. Given that my cancer was advanced, I worried that the side effects would overshadow any benefits I might experience and affect my quality of life. After serious conversations with my doctor, we decided to hold off on chemotherapy for now, leaving the choice open for the future if my situation changed.

When I initially researched chemotherapy, I found it unsurprising that doctors often recommended it, as it proved highly effective for various cancers and helped many patients. But for me, deciding whether to go through with it was a deeply personal choice. While chemotherapy can kill cancer cells and shrink tumors, it also comes with side effects that can significantly affect daily life.

I know everyone's cancer journey is different, and it is important to have honest discussions with your family and doctors. For me, it was about exploring traditional and alternative therapies and finding what feels right. Have you considered potential treatment plans, and which ones would help you the most?

A few days after our meeting with the oncologist, I thought about how I wanted this experience to unfold. The idea of taking it day by day—something I had often heard but rolled my eyes at—struck a chord with me. Each moment felt like an opportunity to learn and grow, shaping my path in unexpected ways.

Living one day at a time might sound simple, but it can be incredibly difficult. It is easy to get caught up in worries about the future, making it hard to stay grounded in the present. Each day brings new trials, and I knew I needed to consciously seek moments of peace and acceptance. This struggle highlighted the importance of self-compassion as I dealt with my feelings and tried to embrace each day, despite the fear that cancer brings.

From my years in business, I learned that when faced with a problem like cancer, you do not just sit there lost in thought. Instead, you actively look for solutions and take steps to implement them.

This made me think about the value of seeking other opinions. I knew some cancer patients felt compelled to get a second or even third opinion after a diagnosis, and that this could be an important part of exploring all available options. In my case, I did not feel it was necessary. However, there are reasons you might want to do so.

Some people seek additional opinions because of uncertainties or doubts about their diagnosis. A friend of mine felt it was worth it because another oncologist might offer a different approach or access to unique clinical trials that his current doctor did not. If your diagnosis is rare, getting a fresh perspective can provide clarity and alternative paths to consider.

If you are feeling uneasy or uncertain, seeking other opinions can help you make informed decisions about your care. Consulting another specialist can also provide reassurance, either confirming your treatment path or opening new possibilities.

It is essential to trust your instincts and advocate for your health, especially on such a critical and personal journey. While I was satisfied with the opinions I had received, I understood this might not be the case for everyone. Have you considered getting a second opinion?

PAUSE FOR THOUGHT

After a cancer diagnosis, choosing the best path forward involves careful consideration of treatment options, lifestyle changes, and emotional support. This process can feel overwhelming, but taking the time to weigh each option can help us take control of our journey. It is essential to engage in conversations with our oncologists and families, exploring all potential therapies to find the best path that aligns with our needs for recovery. Embracing this approach ensures that we are not alone in this fight and reinforces the importance of making informed choices.

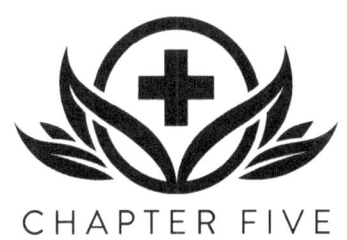

CHAPTER FIVE

Moments of Clarity

I made some tentative decisions. Because I get tired quite easily, my doctor advised against a lot of physical exertion. I crossed off two things I had spent much time on: heavy gardening and 18 holes of golf. It may seem odd, but cutting those two activities brought me more relief than a sense of loss.

Even now, I do not feel cheated out of something, as you might expect. The main point I decided on was to make a positive effort to avoid withdrawing from life. This way, I can develop a supportive environment that encourages my healing and creates a sense of belonging.

There are some immediate issues of the day that require my attention. One of the unseen benefits often found in experiencing a serious illness is the invaluable opportunity to put your house in order—not just in a practical sense, but emotionally and spiritually as well. While I have kept up with the bills, there are some financial matters that need to be addressed.

This can take hours, and my powers of concentration are not at their best, so I can only manage a little every morning. While I am taking care of these matters, I realize I am not thinking about my illness. That is good, I soon decide. When I see that busy work is getting done, there is a feeling of both relief and accomplishment.

It amazed me how cancer had affected my ability to concentrate and focus. Lack of concentration is a frequent problem for individuals facing cancer, often stemming from the physical and emotional toll of the illness and its treatments. To cope with this, I began using a calendar to manage my tasks and appointments, which lessened the pressure of trying to keep everything in my head.

By visualizing my schedule, I could choose what I wanted to do each day and make sure that nothing slipped through the cracks. Breaking tasks into manageable steps allowed me to focus on completing one small job at a time, reducing feelings of frustration.

I quickly learned that multitasking often left my brain feeling cluttered and fatigued, making it difficult to concentrate. By making a list and prioritizing my daily tasks, I maintained focus and made steady progress on what mattered most. Sleep also played a significant role in concentration. After a decent night's rest, my focus improved significantly, enabling me to tackle my daily tasks with greater ease.

A good friend suggested that whenever I noticed my concentration waning, I should take a few minutes to stretch and drink some water, which made a remarkable difference. These simple acts allowed me to return to the task at hand with renewed energy. What have you done to improve your concentration and focus?

Another big step for me was deciding to get dressed. I had spent the last few weeks in my bathrobe and pajamas. The decision to put on "real clothes" each day was a powerful affirmation of life. It represented a small yet meaningful step toward regaining a sense of normalcy and control in a distressing situation.

While it may not seem important, getting dressed helped me re-establish a sense of routine and structure during the turmoil of medical appointments, treatments, and uncertainty. Putting on clothes symbolized my strength and determination to face the day, regardless of the challenges that lay ahead. It also helped boost my mood and self-esteem. Most importantly, putting on clothes helped me feel better about myself, which was something I desperately needed.

Although this was a significant milestone for me, a particularly important development occurred during this time: my wife and I started conversing in ways we hadn't been able to before. Initially, conversations about my illness were too stressful, making it difficult to talk openly. However, we've reached a point where we can discuss my condition more freely.

Often, our conversations feel as if we are discussing a third party or another couple, which allows us to approach the topic with a bit more distance. This perspective helps us navigate our discussions more objectively, benefiting us both. This shift allowed us to express our fears and hopes more freely without feeling overwhelmed by the weight of the situation.

This newfound openness in our communication was further strengthened by the bonds we were building with family and friends. Engaging in these conversations with loved ones brought more layers of support and understanding to our lives. We found that sharing our thoughts and feelings with others not only lightened some emotional burdens but also helped build a sense of community.

It was comforting to know that we were not alone in this journey, as many of our friends and family offered their support in countless ways—whether through listening, sharing their own stories, or simply being present. This created a nurturing environment that helped us both cope with the uncertainty of the future. How have you and your spouse discussed your cancer diagnosis and treatment?

PAUSE FOR THOUGHT

Getting dressed while dealing with cancer can have several benefits, including boosting our moods and creating a sense of normalcy. Wearing clothes we feel comfortable and confident in can help us maintain a positive self-image and motivate us to engage in daily activities. Getting dressed helps combat negative thoughts and feelings associated with our illnesses. Additionally, being able to talk about our disease encourages conversations that can provide hope and encouragement for both ourselves and others.

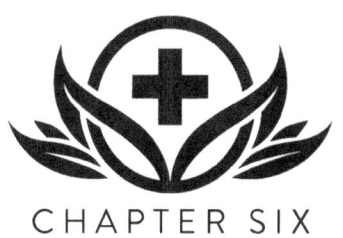

CHAPTER SIX

Dealing with Frustrations

I have never considered myself a religious person, but I have always felt a connection to something more spiritual. While I seldom attended services at our local community church, I enjoyed several rounds of golf with the pastor and found him genuinely likable. Our conversations were always engaging, filled with interesting experiences he shared. So, I reached out to him, expressing my desire to continue our discussions. I believe I was seeking a way to make my peace with God.

One day, he appeared at my house unannounced. I welcomed him in with a nervous smile, hoping to hide my surprise. "Hey, sorry for dropping by without calling first. Checking in seemed like a good idea since I was in the neighborhood," he said.

After a few minutes of small talk, we dove into our conversation. I could not shake the feeling that the pastor was not fully grasping the emotional weight of my situation, and I struggled to follow his words. Perhaps it would have been beneficial for me to take a moment to reflect on what I hoped to gain from our discussion before we began. As our conversation continued, it felt like we were drifting further away from the comfort I was seeking. By the end of nearly two hours, I sensed we were both mentally exhausted.

At this point, I felt a deep sense of disappointment. I could not find consolation through our discussion. Maybe one meeting was not enough, but we did not make plans to get together again. Sometimes, despite good intentions, the suggestions offered by others may not reach deeply enough to provide the support we hope for. Ultimately, finding peace is a deeply personal journey, and it may take time and exploration to discover what truly brings comfort.

My relationship with the pastor on the golf course revolved around friendly competition and genuine camaraderie, which made our time together enjoyable. However, this laid-back dynamic may have made it difficult for him to connect with me during such a serious time. We often focused on fun and friendly competition, which likely made it hard for him to shift to the deeper emotional support I needed. Nevertheless, it was a frustrating experience.

While not directly related, I encountered another frustration the following week. A headline in the newspaper caught my eye. It was news about cancer and a possible research breakthrough. It led me to believe that something good was about to happen; the long-awaited moment might be near.

I read on hurriedly, and as I got into the body of the article, I realized that for my type of lung cancer, it was irrelevant. I could not help but think that some PR person was trying to keep cancer in the headlines so that research funding would continue to be available.

Again, a few days later, I heard a human-interest story on TV about a "cancer remedy," where a woman had defied all odds and achieved an incredible recovery. It made me wonder if something similar could happen to me, causing a moment of hope mixed with skepticism about claims that often seemed too good to be true.

A well-meaning friend told me about an acquaintance who had been helped in Mexico by a new, innovative treatment. "What have you got to lose?" he asked. Another friend suggested a clinic in New York and mentioned their success with cancer patients. I wondered if they could do anything for me that my doctors here could not do. I seriously doubted it and pushed these ideas out of my mind. At this point, I was physically unable to venture off to some distant place in search of a miracle.

However, my strong interest in finding an effective treatment led me to consider all options. Talking openly with my oncologist helped me distinguish what was realistically possible for my illness and how to determine genuine possibilities from false hopes.

I feel confident my doctor is better prepared to handle my specific type of cancer and its complications than any doctors I might find elsewhere. I wondered if pursuing these options would add to or detract from that goal. I concluded that they would detract. I finally decided to set aside those choices.

With this understanding, I investigated various treatments that could lessen discomfort, such as pain management therapies, nutritional support, and integrative approaches like acupuncture and meditation. The knowledge that I was actively participating in my care and making informed choices helped me further improve my quality of life.

I found joy in the little moments—sharing laughter with friends, enjoying my favorite meals, or taking a leisurely walk. By redirecting my energy toward improving my physical and emotional health, I discovered a renewed sense of hope and purpose to guide me through each day. How do you handle stories that seem like believable remedies for cancer but you know are too good to be true?

PAUSE FOR THOUGHT

Hope often shines brightly during difficult times, increasing our desire for healing and a future filled with possibilities. Yet, frustrations can arise from what we read and hear about potential cures, the uncertainty of the experience, and the emotional toll of treatment. In these moments, it's essential to develop patience and focus on the small accomplishments that help us keep moving forward. Celebrating these victories—whether it's a good day or simply managing to get out of bed—reminds us that progress is still possible, even when the journey feels daunting.

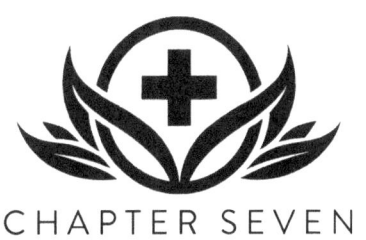

CHAPTER SEVEN

Dark Thoughts

Facing cancer can stir up many emotions, including dark thoughts that often creep in during quiet moments of the day or night. It is important to accept these feelings, as they are a natural response to an incredibly life-altering disease. My own dark thoughts often arose from a deep-seated fear of the unknown and worries about how my illness would affect my loved ones. Accepting these feelings was essential on my journey.

Dealing with cancer can lead to unpredictable emotional ups and downs, often characterized by intense feelings and rapid mood shifts. You might experience joy and excitement one moment, followed by sadness or anxiety the next, creating a turbulent emotional experience.

You may feel hopeful after a good visit with your oncologist and then feel disappointment as you struggle with the unpredictability of symptoms and treatment responses. Adjusting to these changes is not easy and often brings a sense of loss—not just of health, but of the life you once knew.

Managing treatments while confronting the harsh realities of your illness can lead to frustration. It is a path that most would like to avoid, yet it is a reality faced by countless individuals and their families. Recognizing these difficult emotions and seeking help—from friends, family, or cancer therapists—is important for feeling better and less stressed during this period. Cancer and depression often go hand in hand. Although I never experienced severe depression, many people do.

If you are feeling depressed, seek help from a mental health professional or a support group; they can offer comfort and guidance through your complex emotions. Ultimately, taking proactive steps to care for your mental health is just as important as addressing your physical health. Never ignore depression; it is a significant issue!

On days when I felt low, I redirected my focus to activities I enjoyed that helped lift my spirits. Setting achievable, short-term goals provided a sense of purpose and accomplishment. This could be anything from watering the garden, working on a puzzle, or taking an online course that interests you.

Small achievements helped change my perspective. I also reflected on what had given my life meaning. Writing down my thoughts became a valuable way to process my emotions and find purpose in my experience.

When I discussed dark thoughts with a friend, he emphasized how important exercise had been for him during his cancer journey. "Even in small amounts, exercise provided significant benefits. I found that activities like walking or stretching helped reduce symptoms like fatigue and anxiety while also improving flexibility."

Sometimes, the most powerful opponent you will ever face stares back at you in the mirror, reflecting the internal battle you may be experiencing.

It emphasizes that, while cancer is an external enemy, the true struggle often lies within us—our thoughts, fears, doubts, and emotions.

The mirror can serve as a reminder of the reality of your illness and your fight against it. This can bring feelings of vulnerability and even despair. The reflection symbolizes not only the physical changes brought on by cancer and its treatments but also the mental strength needed to cope with the challenges ahead.

This internal conflict can be just as threatening as the physical challenges caused by the disease as we struggle with feelings of uncertainty about the future. Recognizing this internal battle is essential, as it allows us to confront these fears directly, helping us seek the support we need and find strength in our vulnerability.

As cancer patients, we must remember we are not alone in this experience; together, we can face the emotional realities of this disease and offer support and understanding to one another along the way. Our shared journey increases our determination and encourages hope.

As I consider these heavy emotions, I also hold on to the ordinary parts of life that still exist. For me, writing letters has always been an important way to connect. Every year, I would send out a Christmas letter to my family and friends, sharing updates and joy. During my illness, I have been fortunate to receive many warm letters, notes, and get-well cards that have truly brightened my days.

Two letters from my sister Florence stand out. The first was about a project focused on our childhood experiences; she included a set of questions for me to answer. When I received her letter, I did not respond right away. After she learned about my illness, she quickly reached out again, apologizing for her earlier letter and encouraging me to disregard it. She did not want to add to my stress by making me feel obligated to answer her questions.

However, since I was genuinely interested in the subject, I wrote back and explained my delay. In my response, I opened up about my thoughts on my illness, admitting that I had considered going to bed and pulling the covers over my head. Again, I realized something important: I had a choice. I could either give in to despair or explore different options to move forward.

This realization led me to a powerful conclusion: I want to engage with life, even in the face of unpredictability. This decision opened the door to a more meaningful existence in the months that followed. Acceptance of this possibility has filled my journey with hope and connection, reminding me that even in the darkest moments, there can be light.

PAUSE FOR THOUGHT

Cancer can cast a shadow of dark thoughts as fear and uncertainty creep in, questioning our sense of control and well-being. Accepting these feelings and seeking support allows us to deal with our emotions, creating a more hopeful outlook for the journey ahead. This resilience can transform our experience, encouraging personal growth and deeper relationships with loved ones. By acknowledging our vulnerabilities and sharing our fears with those we trust, we open the door to healing connections and find comfort in knowing we are not alone in this fight.

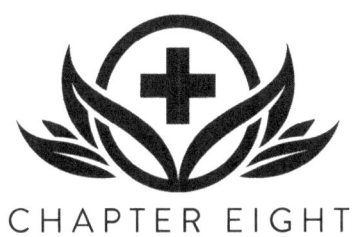

CHAPTER EIGHT

Embracing Change

My wife and I have begun an inspiring journey of transformation, planting seeds of change that promise to grow within us. As we cultivate these new ideas and beliefs, we recognize the importance of integrating them into our daily lives. Rather than allowing them to remain mere thoughts, we want to develop a meaningful philosophy that rings true with our experiences.

At first, it may seem simple, but we know that real change can be complicated. Take learning to play tennis, for example. While reading the rules and discussing strategies is valuable, true mastery comes from dedicating time on the court, applying what you've learned through practice. This practice is essential as we work on changing our mindset.

As we go through this new phase in our lives, we often feel confused and unsure, especially when it comes to social plans. Maybe you've hesitated about attending a family gathering or dinner with friends, not knowing how you will feel that day. These feelings are normal and usually arise from wanting to take care of our emotional and physical health—especially when facing challenges like cancer, which can change how we feel from hour to hour or day to day.

By recognizing these feelings, we can make better decisions about our social commitments, only agreeing to things I know I can handle. This uncertainty can be tough and may shake our confidence about the future.

But what if we viewed these moments of hesitation as chances to learn about ourselves and set healthy boundaries? Instead of seeing uncertainty as a roadblock, we can see it as a chance for self-discovery and growth. This perspective helps us understand our needs better and encourages healthier relationships through clearer communication.

I remember my doctor's wise advice when I asked for guidance: "Focus on small achievements, cherish joyful moments, and don't hesitate to ask for help." This perspective truly changed how I view things. I realized that the purpose of this journey may not be a grand destination but rather the process itself—full of learning, connection, and the resilience to keep moving forward.

This shift in thinking became even more meaningful during a conversation with friends who had also faced the challenges of cancer. As we shared our experiences, we found ourselves considering a compelling question: Why does cancer create such a fear in people compared to other illnesses?

We recognized that this fear is understandable—A diagnosis often brings uncertainty about the prognosis. The varied nature of the disease, various stages, and treatment responses can lead to unpredictable outcomes, making it challenging for patients and their families to cope.

It is also essential to be aware of the news we consume and the conversations we engage in; surrounding ourselves with positive influences can significantly improve our outlook. Whether it is connecting with uplifting friends or looking for inspiring stories, these little shifts can profoundly change our perspective, helping us cultivate resilience and find hope during life's difficulties.

Amid these concerns about negative influences, it is important to recognize that advancements in research and treatment have changed many outcomes. By focusing on the progress in cancer care, we can find strength and hope in our experiences. While cancer presents its challenges, we have more tools and support at our disposal than ever before.

As we move forward, let us focus on actively improving our mental health and building courage and hope. Together, we can navigate this time of change and emerge stronger on the other side. Let's celebrate the small wins, support one another, and remember that even in the face of uncertainty, there is a community ready to lift us up.

A friend shared this story with me when his wife was dealing with cancer a few years ago: "Facing my wife's illness brought us closer together. The vulnerability and rawness of dealing with something like cancer stripped away the usual distractions. In our case, the illness created an environment where communication became more open, and we learned to lean on each other in new and profound ways. We also appreciated the small moments, the quiet acts of care, and the strength that came from simply being present for one another."

His words provided me with another reason to feel optimistic!

PAUSE FOR THOUGHT

The diagnosis of cancer can act as a powerful seed of change, prompting us to rethink our priorities and genuinely appreciate life's fleeting moments. As this seed takes root, it can inspire personal growth, encourage meaningful relationships, and begin a renewed commitment to living with purpose and intention. It reminds us to treasure each day and the opportunities it brings. Embracing this newfound perspective allows us to find joy in simple experiences, changing our outlook and motivating us to create lasting memories with those we love.

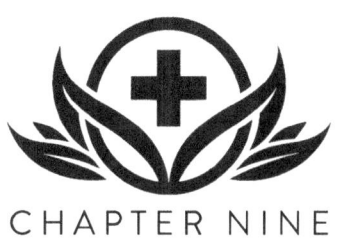

CHAPTER NINE

Family Time

Today, our son came for a visit, and we had a great afternoon together. I wasn't entirely ready to dive into a deep discussion about my cancer, even though we had spoken on the phone several times since my diagnosis. So, we went outside and enjoyed a warm day while watching golfers on the 13th hole of the golf course, just steps away from our patio. The peaceful surroundings helped create a calm atmosphere between us.

I could tell there were questions he wanted to ask, but I appreciated our unspoken understanding that there would be plenty of time for those conversations in the future. For now, we simply enjoyed each other's company, sharing light-hearted stories and reminiscing about happier times.

This visit marked the beginning of a weekly tradition I eagerly looked forward to. It became a source of strength and comfort for me as I navigated this challenging journey. Our son's presence brought a sense of normalcy that I desperately needed, reminding me that even in uncertainty, there are beautiful days to cherish and meaningful connections to nurture.

Another uplifting event was when our daughter flew in from Denver for a long weekend with her two older children. My wife and I eagerly anticipated their arrival, though I had some reservations. Would I be able to manage the trip to the airport? Would I be able to handle the energy, noise, and activity that would undoubtedly fill our home? Fortunately, our friends stepped in to help with coordination, easing my worries about the airport.

The energy of their visit shook us out of our routines and lifted our spirits, breaking the monotony that had settled in. By the end of the weekend, my wife and I noticed a wonderful shift in our attitudes. It felt like a turning point! I found myself more open to embracing a positive approach to the difficulties posed by my illness. This visit reminded me of the joy that family brings and reignited a sense of hope I had been struggling to maintain.

Talking with family and close friends about my illness was emotionally draining, yet encouraging open communication is vital for getting support during such a tough time. I found that creating a comfortable space, free from distractions, for our conversation helped set the stage for sharing feelings and thoughts. It is important to discuss your diagnosis clearly and what it means for your health, as this lays the groundwork for an honest conversation.

I encouraged my family and friends to share their thoughts and feelings. By asking questions like, "How do you feel about this?" or "What concerns do you have?" I wanted us to have a two-way conversation that helped us all process our emotions together.

This approach not only allowed them to express their fears but also reinforced the sense of unity and support within our relationships. Creating an environment where everyone feels included and heard can strengthen bonds and provide mutual comfort during uncertainty. Do you have specific ideas about how you can begin this conversation with your family and friends?

It is necessary to take a different approach when discussing a serious illness like cancer with younger children. You want to make sure you use simple, clear language. For example, I might say, "I am very sick, and the doctors don't know when I will get better."

This straightforward approach ensures that children understand the situation without being confused by complex medical terms. Encouraging them to ask questions is important, and it's normal for them to repeat the same questions as they take in the information.

Along with open communication, I suggested my grandchildren create memories with me—like making a scrapbook. Doing an activity like this helps them feel connected and provides something for them to hold on to in the future. Letting them know it is okay to continue pursuing their interests and finding happiness, even while I am sick, is vital.

It reassures them that life can still be meaningful despite difficult circumstances. Encouraging an open conversation about their feelings—whether they are sad or confused—helps create a deeper bond as we experience this time together. Can you think of any activities you could do with your children or grandchildren to create memories together?

PAUSE FOR THOUGHT

Family visits can offer emotional support and a sense of comfort during times of illness. Sharing our experiences and feelings with loved ones can be difficult, but it encourages deeper relationships and understanding, allowing us to focus on recovery. These visits can create special moments of love and laughter, lifting our spirits and promoting a positive outlook during this time. Additionally, the presence of family can serve as a reminder of the strength we possess, reinforcing our determination to face the challenges ahead with courage and hope.

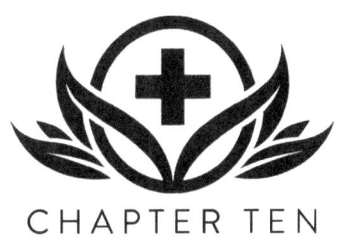

CHAPTER TEN

A New Perspective

I would not describe myself as religious, but my parents raised me in a deeply religious household as the second youngest of twelve children. Growing up in such a large family, faith was a significant part of our daily lives, shaping our values and interactions.

One memory that often comes to mind is of my brother, Sam. After dedicating many years as a missionary in India, he returned home aged and disabled. With his wife having passed away and no money to speak of, Sam found himself in a small home for elderly church workers in Ohio.

On a visit not long ago, my wife asked Sam, "How do you like it here?" He paused for a moment, lost in thought. Then, with a gentle smile spreading across his face, he replied, "I must quote a scripture: The Apostle Paul once wrote, 'For I have learned to be content regardless of the circumstances.'" His words carried deep meaning, reflecting a philosophy that went beyond his unusual situation.

Sam's ability to find contentment in such basic circumstances was a powerful lesson in strength and perspective. His unwavering appreciation for the little things inspired me to rethink my own definition of contentment. I wondered why we so often chase after comforts, believing they will bring us happiness.

His positive spirit in the face of adversity inspired me to adopt a similar outlook during my own struggles. In a world where material possessions often dictate our happiness, Sam's wisdom reminds us of the strength found in acceptance and gratitude.

As I continued my journey with cancer, I often wondered: If you are not religious but more spiritual, is dealing with a cancer diagnosis more difficult? I found that the experience can vary from person to person.

For me, my spirituality has played a significant role in helping me find meaning in my experiences, including my illness. It provides a lens through which I can navigate the emotional complexities of cancer, allowing me to find a sense of purpose even in the face of adversity.

In moments of uncertainty and fear, I find comfort in connecting with the beauty that surrounds me—whether through nature or the simple joys of daily life. Spending quiet time reflecting and even praying has become an essential practice that grounds me, offering comfort as I work through my feelings about my illness.

While some may find it more difficult to navigate their cancer without a religious framework, I have discovered that my spiritual beliefs provide a solid foundation during this tough time.

This sense of spirituality has allowed me to build resilience, encouraging me to focus on the lessons and growth that can come from this experience. It helps me develop an attitude of gratitude, allowing me to appreciate the support of loved ones, the beauty of small moments, and the strength I did not realize I had. Have you ever noticed how changing your perspective can shift your entire experience?

Thinking back on my visit with Sam, I realize it inspired a real change in my outlook. Did the memory of that visit help me further accept my cancer diagnosis? Absolutely. It helped me see my illness as an integral part of my life journey rather than just a source of suffering. This shift brought a deep sense of peace and clarity that I had long sought.

Embracing cancer does not mean giving up or losing hope; instead, it represents a brave choice to face reality while living fully during the challenges. I understand that acknowledging my illness can coexist with a hopeful outlook, promoting resilience and strength.

Each person's journey toward acceptance is unique, and it is important to approach this process with compassion and kindness—for ourselves and others. We all cope in our own ways, and recognizing this can create a supportive environment for healing and connection.

By accepting both our struggles and our hopes, we can find moments of joy and meaning even in the most difficult times. I understand this experience is not just about facing my illness but also about celebrating life and the connections I share with those I love.

As I reflect on my brother's strength and the lessons I have learned, I feel a renewed sense of purpose. How can I carry these insights forward and inspire others who may be facing their own challenges?

I hope to share the strength I've gained from my experiences, reminding others that even in the darkest moments, there is always a light to guide us. How can you make your cancer journey inspire others fighting a similar battle?

PAUSE FOR THOUGHT

Finding contentment in tough times requires us to develop an attitude that embraces appreciation and mindfulness, focusing on the small joys that can still be found each day. By recognizing our feelings and intentionally seeking moments of peace and happiness, we can create a sense of stability and fulfillment, even during this difficult experience. Expressing appreciation for even the simplest pleasures—a warm cup of tea, a beautiful sunset, or a comforting conversation—can help shift our perspective and nurture a deeper sense of inner peace amid the chaos.

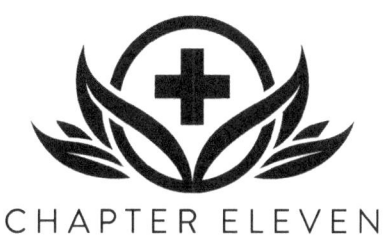

CHAPTER ELEVEN

Soul Searching

Throughout my life, I have always been interested in national and international events, closely following global issues and crises. However, after my diagnosis, topics that once captivated me, like economic uncertainty, suddenly felt trivial. I thought, "Do ongoing conflicts, such as those in the Middle East, really need my input right now?" Questions about the president's stance on various issues seemed increasingly irrelevant.

It made me wonder how often I find myself caught up in the world's problems, only to realize I have my own significant challenges to face, which occupy much of my mental and emotional space. Losing interest in current affairs is a common experience for someone dealing with cancer; the stress and anxiety surrounding a diagnosis can feel all-consuming.

My ability to concentrate on complex topics diminished significantly during this time. Instead of diving into heavy news, I turned to lighter shows that provided a welcome distraction— feel-good movies, light-hearted TV series, or a program on National Geographic.

To strike a balance, I decided that one news show in the evening was enough, which helped me stay informed without feeling overloaded. This routine gave structure to my day while allowing me to focus on uplifting content that lightened my mood.

This shift in focus made me aware of another common pattern among those facing cancer: unintentionally building barriers between ourselves and others. If it were not for my friends' persistent efforts to reach out, I might have completely retreated into my own bubble. While I didn't want to isolate myself, I discovered that connecting and conversing with friends was an enjoyable way to stay informed. I found this preferable to relying solely on the often-negative media.

Something else happened. I felt a strong need to confront the reality of my circumstances. I had previously assured myself that I was untroubled by the unknown, yet as I dug deeper into my thoughts, I knew this was not entirely true. I worried about the unpredictability of treatments, the physical and emotional toll they could take, and the potential strain on my relationships and daily routines.

Recognizing and accepting these emotions became important, as it allowed me to deal with the complexities of my situation rather than push them aside. This perspective not only helped me bounce back from setbacks but also motivated me to continue to grow.

When I embraced my vulnerabilities, I confronted my fears and uncertainties head-on. This process helped to lessen my anxiety, making future challenges feel more manageable. Have you ever discovered that confronting your fears can lead to unexpected avenues of personal growth?

When faced with life's fragility, my wife and I found ourselves treasuring our time together. This led to a renewed sense of partnership, one built not just on the everyday routines of life but on a mutual commitment to support each other through the most frustrating periods. While my illness presented its challenges, it also created a sense of resilience in our marriage that carried us forward with even greater strength and understanding.

In my soul-searching, I have come to realize that reflection is not just about finding answers but about embracing the questions. How do I want to spend my time? What can I learn from this experience? As I consider these things, I feel a deep change within me. Vulnerability has become a powerful incentive for growth. It's in these moments of openness that I discover that strength lies not in the absence of fear, but in the willingness to face it.

As I reflect on my experiences, I recognize the importance of connection. Sharing my thoughts and feelings with others creates bonds that enrich my life. Every interaction brings a new insight, and each shared story adds to my understanding. Instead of seeking immediate solutions, I am allowing myself to sit with the discomfort of uncertainty. In doing so, I realize that every question I embrace leads me further along my path.

Cultivating bravery can help you navigate this tough time. Start by acknowledging your feelings; it is normal to experience fear, anger, and disappointment. Educate yourself about your diagnosis and treatment options to help you make informed decisions. Build a trusting relationship with your doctors, as open communication can ease fears and provide clarity.

And most importantly, continue to hope for positive outcomes, through both treatment and appreciating everyday moments, as bravery is about facing fears and continuing to move forward despite them. Each brave decision, no matter how small, builds your strength and helps you reclaim a sense of control in the face of adversity.

PAUSE FOR THOUGHT

Self-reflection encourages us to dig into our lives, helping us confront what really matters. In this process, we learn that being vulnerable and open are essential qualities that can lead us to a better understanding of ourselves, our relationships with others, and what it means to truly live. It also helps us become more aware of our thoughts, feelings, and behaviors and how they affect our recovery. This journey of introspection creates personal growth and resilience as we navigate our challenges.

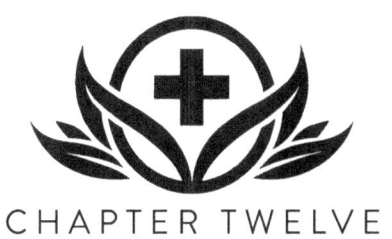

CHAPTER TWELVE

A Silver Lining

It is quite common for individuals diagnosed with cancer to experience feelings of victimization. These feelings can stem from the perception of losing control over your body and health, as well as the social and emotional repercussions of the illness. They can also be part of the grieving process for the life you had before your cancer.

Identifying as a victim often leads to a cycle of self-pity and helplessness. I knew that such an attitude would cloud my judgment and hinder my ability to move forward. During this period, I responded by rejecting the word "victim." I am not a victim, nor do I see myself that way. This became a red flag for me whenever I heard the term.

My rejection of the word "victim" became a path toward personal growth. I learned that while we cannot always control the circumstances that life throws our way, we can control how we respond to them. I began to build an attitude that was not defined by my difficulties but strengthened by my ability to overcome them.

It is important for individuals experiencing these feelings to have support, whether through friends, family, support groups, or mental health professionals. Talking openly about these emotions can be helpful in processing them and finding ways to cope.

I also discovered a silver lining: my family and friends continued to see me as an active participant in society, valuing my thoughts and contributions. They treated me not merely as someone defined by illness but as a person with insights, experiences, and a voice that mattered. Their unwavering support reminded me that my identity went beyond my illness; it was rooted in the relationships I treasured and the impact I could still make in their lives.

It was a powerful reminder that, despite the physical and emotional difficulties I faced, I could still engage meaningfully with the world around me and that my presence could bring comfort and inspiration to others as well. What is your silver lining?

I was fortunate that this victim mentality did not last long. However, I was very aware that my gradual withdrawal from the world had placed a burden on my wife. Although she had adjusted to this change with remarkable grace, I could see that she missed the social interactions that had once been a big part of our lives together.

To help her feel included, I made a conscious decision to engage more with others, taking part in activities that promoted connection and camaraderie. I approached this in a fairly normal way. Much like learning how to walk again, which involves a few tentative first steps, the journey of rediscovering life—possibly in a new light—starts with small, intentional actions.

One of those actions stemmed from my passion for reading; a thoughtful friend recognized this and lent me a copy of a book dedicated to navigating the challenges of coping with cancer. However, as I dove into its pages, I found that the experiences it described felt distant from my own, leaving me to look for something that more closely mirrored my story.

Despite the well-meaning intentions behind my friend's suggestion, I was looking for books that acknowledged the complexities of my journey—stories that explored the emotional aspects of living with cancer rather than simply offering coping strategies. Other friends shared more books with me, but many of them felt superficial. Now I reflect on how little I knew about this world of cancer before my diagnosis threw me into this frightening experience.

It became clear that dealing with this disease required more than just reading words on a page; I needed something that would help me grasp the realities that went beyond what these guides offered. Maybe there were not many good books out there on the subject of cancer! I guess I should consider writing my own!

I wondered how I could focus on improving my well-being today to create positive moments for tomorrow, despite my illness and uncertain future. Slowly, I discovered that for some time, it would involve living as usual.

Yes, there would be some changes. No, I would not be playing 18 holes of golf today. Yes, I would get up, get dressed, eat breakfast, and try to follow a daily schedule. Not a rigid one, of course, but a flexible plan. This routine not only provided structure to my day but also helped me maintain a positive outlook, as I understood just how important that could be.

I have always been fairly optimistic, but with cancer, that is not always easy. So, I dug into some research on the topic. It is incredible to see how having a hopeful outlook can significantly influence cancer patients. It's not just about feeling better mentally; it can also have a positive impact on our physical health.

I came across studies suggesting that those who maintain an optimistic view of their condition usually have lower stress levels. And let's face it, stress is not great for anyone, especially when battling something like cancer! Plus, when we adopt a more upbeat attitude, we are more likely to engage in healthier habits and build a solid support network, which can significantly affect survival rates.

But let's be honest: staying positive throughout a cancer journey is not always easy. There are days when the weight of it all feels like too much. It is tough not to be swept away by fear, sadness, or uncertainty about what the future holds. Some days, forcing on a brave face feels like just another chore on an already loaded plate.

That said, I have found that a positive outlook can be a lifeline. While it cannot cure cancer, it helps us cope, manage treatments, and look for meaning in our experiences. Interestingly, when I try to stay optimistic, I notice my friends and family respond positively as well. My attitude creates an uplifting vibe that encourages healing and connection all around. What strategies do you use to keep your spirits up?

PAUSE FOR THOUGHT

The range of emotions we encounter during a cancer journey can be overwhelming, taking us from fear and anger to moments of hope and joy. This emotional experience is a natural response to the challenges faced. Optimism creates a supportive environment that improves our immune system and our overall quality of life. By developing a positive attitude, we can better navigate the complexities of treatment and find meaning in our experiences. Embracing this emotional journey can help us live more fully and build a foundation for healing.

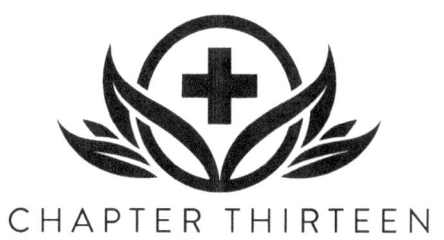

CHAPTER THIRTEEN

Whirlwind of Emotions

Physically, I have experienced some minor discomfort, but most days I have felt more energetic and better than expected. I see my oncologist every few weeks, and he always opens our conversation with the question, "Well, how are you feeling?"

In order to be as helpful as possible, I tried to plan out my answer in advance. This time, I concluded that I felt ambivalent. I thought it was a good word, but I questioned its appropriateness in this instance. Looking it up later convinced me it perfectly described how I felt.

The word "ambivalent" captured my feelings when the doctor asked how I was doing. Receiving my cancer diagnosis left me feeling caught in a whirlwind of emotions. On one hand, there is a profound sense of fear and uncertainty about the future, leading to anxiety and sadness. The weight of not knowing what lies ahead can feel suffocating as I deal with the realities of treatment, potential side effects, and the impact on my loved ones.

On the other hand, this dual awareness encourages me to navigate the path ahead with grace and strength, reinforcing that I am more than my illness. While cancer is a part of my story, it does not define the life I want to live. I have discovered that it is okay to feel conflicted and to experience joy even during a difficult time.

But I also know that facing a serious illness can lead you to question who you are. When cancer enters the picture, it often disrupts your daily life, routines, and future plans. You may find it hard to align your sense of self —defined by your jobs, activities, and dreams — with your new reality as someone with cancer. The fear of what might happen can push you to think deeply about what really matters in your life.

Cancer treatments can bring both noticeable and subtle changes to your body, such as losing weight, hair, or energy. These changes can affect how you see yourself and how you believe others see you. If you have always found a sense of identity in your role, such as being a teacher or a lawyer, a cancer diagnosis can shift this role, leaving you feeling lost or uncertain about your purpose.

Social relationships can also change dramatically. Friends and family may not know what to say or do, which can make you feel lonely or misunderstood. This can lead to doubts about your place in your social circles. The emotional burden of cancer can bring feelings of sadness and fear, which may cause you to question your own strength and ability to cope.

On the flip side, I have discovered strengths I never realized I had. This newfound courage has led me to redefine who I am based on my experience. The label of "cancer patient" can feel heavy, and I am torn between seeing myself as a patient and remembering the person I was before the diagnosis.

Cancer can also spark significant questions about life, purpose, and what it means to truly live well. This deep thinking can challenge long-held beliefs and values. In searching for ways to cope with your illness, you may explore various aspects of your identity, including spiritual beliefs, personal interests, or creative outlets, prompting a reevaluation of who you are and what brings you happiness.

Recognizing this, I have found that the road to recovery is rarely a straight line; it is more like the fluctuations of a weather pattern. For instance, spring does not offer a consistent march toward warmer days but rather a mix of warmth interspersed with unexpected cold snaps.

I have come to expect these ups and downs; after enjoying good days, setbacks can feel even more intense. Healing is not just physical; it is a multifaceted journey requiring emotional and mental resilience.

I accept the conflicting forces within me and appreciate how they balance each other out—at least for now. It is common to have doubts about my illness, especially when I feel relatively well. I sometimes wonder, "Could the doctors have made a mistake? Is my cancer not as serious after all?"

These fleeting thoughts serve as a coping mechanism, helping me reconcile my outward appearance with the reality of my condition. This desire to align my physical well-being with my emotional state brings moments of hope that the diagnosis is not as severe as it seems.

These moments of self-assurance also offer brief escapes from the weight of this disease, allowing me to experience a sense of normalcy and control. However, it is essential to remember that a diagnosis is based on clinical evaluations and tests; feeling good does not mean that the cancer is gone or that the battle is over. Have you ever questioned your doctor's diagnosis in your own mind?

PAUSE FOR THOUGHT

While we cannot rely on hope alone, it encourages us to imagine a brighter future, inspiring strength during difficult times. Acceptance allows us to embrace our current reality, take positive actions, and welcome the peace that enables us to find meaning during this uncertainty. Together, hope and acceptance become powerful forces on our journey of healing. By integrating these two elements into our lives, we can create a sense of balance that allows us to face each day with courage and purpose.

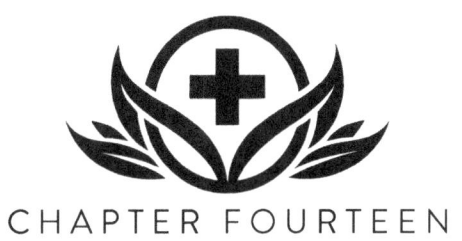

CHAPTER FOURTEEN

Shifting Responsibilities

While I concentrate on living in the present, I am committed to making sure that Marion has everything she needs for the future. I encourage her to stay involved in activities she enjoys, such as going out to lunch with friends, participating in her lecture group, and playing golf.

Starting with plans that do not involve me feels a bit foreign to her, and I understand that stepping outside her comfort zone can be intimidating. But I gently urge her to take these steps, believing that strengthening her independence will allow her to navigate life with even greater confidence.

We have learned to discuss these changes openly, sharing both our concerns and hopes, and even finding moments to laugh about the challenges ahead. This lightheartedness helps ease the weight of our conversations and reinforces our bond as we face this new chapter together.

As we adapt to this growing reality, my wife will need to take on more responsibility regarding our family's business affairs. While she has not always felt confident in this area, I reassure her that she is more than capable.

While I can handle most of these matters on my own perfectly well now, I want her to feel more secure with investments and financial areas she has chosen not to actively engage with in the past. I believe these small steps will help her feel more relaxed with these added commitments.

I have traditionally been the one to organize social activities with friends, and I want her to take the initiative in this area as well. Encouraging her to reach out and connect with others not only prepares her for future social engagements but also opens the door for her to build her own support network.

I have also been the primary gardener in our family, but I know I can no longer keep up with that role. I would like her to take on this responsibility, with a professional gardener assisting with the more difficult projects. I will be here to supervise and provide help. This is not about passing off chores; it is about giving her the chance to create a space she can nurture and enjoy. She loves pulling weeds and clearing away dead flowers, so I believe this chore will be perfect for her!

I had to carefully consider how to shift some responsibilities to my wife without further stressing her out. I started talking about the changes we were facing, sharing my feelings and concerns, and encouraging her to do the same. Having these honest conversations helped us both understand each other's perspectives and created a sense of teamwork as we navigated this new reality together.

Beyond our discussions, I tried to support her wherever I could, even if it was just being there to talk through plans or help with specific tasks. I wanted her to feel supported, not overwhelmed by all the changes happening around us. I shared essential information about bills, appliance warranties, and other household matters, hoping to make her feel as comfortable as possible.

On another subject entirely, I mentioned earlier that my appetite for a while was fragile. Thankfully, that changed! Much of the turning point came from the food my wife cooked for me. She has always been a great cook, and her willingness to cater to my cravings made a significant difference in my recovery. When she asked me what I might enjoy eating, I often thought of simple comfort foods you would not find in any gourmet cookbook.

Surprisingly, these basic but delicious meals became incredibly appealing to me, and before I knew it, they would appear on the table. This personalized touch to my meals helped rekindle my interest in food, and even though I ate small portions at first, it was a step in the right direction. Although my appetite did not return at once, each meal made me feel a little better, both physically and emotionally. What food has particular appeal to you?

Besides the well-prepared meals, I added a little more exercise to my routine. Even something as simple as walking a little farther in the neighborhood or stretching a bit more helped shift my mind to more pleasant thoughts and encouraged me to eat. The movement not only energized me but also created a sense of normalcy amid the difficulties of my illness. As I regained some weight back, I felt a glimmer of hope.

Yet, along with that hope came the nagging worry that my lack of appetite, much like the disease itself, could return at any moment. This realization served as a reminder of the fragility of my situation but also motivated me to continue focusing on my health and well-being. By combining healthy meals with simple exercises, I was slowly reclaiming a sense of control over my body and life, reinforcing the idea that small steps could lead to meaningful progress in my recovery journey.

PAUSE FOR THOUGHT

Preparing our spouses to take on more responsibilities involves talking openly about our hopes and concerns, making them feel supported and informed. By discussing practical matters and encouraging their confidence, we can work together to plan ahead. Flexibility is key, as roles may need to shift depending on circumstances. Regularly checking in with each other about how things are going allows for adjustments when needed. This open communication establishes a sense of teamwork that can strengthen our relationship during difficult times.

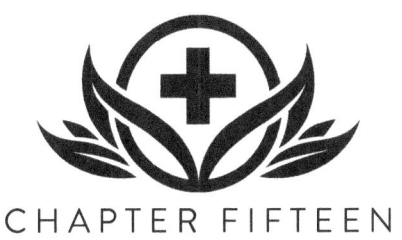

CHAPTER FIFTEEN

Finding Balance

Creating a schedule has become more important than ever for me. I am not exactly a morning person who jumps out of bed ready to tackle the day. However, if there is something planned that I really want to do, I often find that I forget about the effort it takes to get started.

There have been countless early mornings in my life when I eagerly hopped out of bed for a pre-dawn fishing trip or an early tee time. Now, knowing that something fun is scheduled for the day can motivate me to get moving sooner than I might otherwise.

I remind myself that having a schedule of things to do is a good thing, thus keeping my mind away from more immediate problems. Can I keep it up? Who knows? But if I take it one day at a time and I managed to get through yesterday, chances are I can likely get through today. I will let tomorrow worry about itself. Anyway, I have my hands full with today!

Establishing a routine provides several significant benefits. One of the primary advantages is the consistency of care. A regular schedule helps ensure that my medications, treatments, and appointments are not overlooked. Knowing what to expect each day creates a sense of stability that positively affects my mental health.

I also plan time for rest and relaxation. Additionally, this routine encourages social opportunities by scheduling time for family and friends. These social connections are important for emotional support and can enhance my overall quality of life.

Structuring my day around these commitments helps me feel more in control and gives me a clearer sense of purpose. Including small, manageable tasks—like some chair exercises, working on a minor home project, or engaging in a hobby — boosts my sense of accomplishment and provides moments of enjoyment.

Flexibility is key when setting up a schedule, especially since my energy levels and mood can change from day to day. I have learned to listen to my body and adjust my plans accordingly. I try to leave room for spontaneity—if I'm feeling good, I might take the chance to go on a day trip or invite a friend to a lecture on a subject of interest to both of us.

Sometimes, I swap out my usual routines for something more enjoyable, like grabbing a hamburger for lunch with a friend. Even though playing just three or four holes of golf isn't a full round, it's still a fun and fulfilling experience. I view activities differently now than I did not so long ago; every experience feels more precious and meaningful.

Marion and I continue to be able to talk more about my disease. This open discussion has allowed us to explore our feelings and fears without reservation. By normalizing these talks, we've created a safe space where both of us can express our concerns and questions. It has become a valuable outlet for processing the emotional weight of my illness. I find this shift in attitude not only eases my own anxiety but also helps my wife feel more comfortable sharing her thoughts.

Additionally, discussing my cancer has encouraged us to develop coping strategies together. Whether it's planning for upcoming treatments or discussing how to manage side effects, our conversations enable us to work together to find solutions that benefit both of us. We are facing the same fight, with individual and shared challenges. As we try to help each other, we draw closer together. The proximity of a break in our long relationship makes us conscious of what we may be losing.

Mixed with the positives, there are certainly some tough moments and days ahead. While I understand that significant improvement may be unlikely without a remission, I also recognize that I have the strength to face what lies ahead. What more can I hope for? Perhaps not much, but I'm committed to sticking with the routine that has brought us this far, embracing each day with a sense of purpose and determination.

On another note, I can't emphasize enough how important laughter has been during this experience. It's taught me to search for those light moments, even when things feel heavy. Reflecting on good times has also been a meaningful practice for me. Living a relatively normal life with my family boosts not just my well-being but theirs as well.

We have close friends who love to stop by, and their presence always lifts my spirits. They are funny, and the laughter is contagious when they're around. Throughout this tough time, laughter has become a source of comfort and resilience for me. It's been a powerful way to cope, offering me brief escapes from the emotional weight of my illness. These moments of humor have helped me step back and find joy, even during challenges. Laughter has encouraged me to celebrate life and all its difficulties, no matter what I'm facing.

I have found that laughter can change my perspective, so I try to approach my disease with a sense of humor. Finding the funny things in certain experiences—like wearing a T-shirt that says, "Cancer picked the wrong guy to mess with!" or a joke my friend told me about a doctor's waiting room: "Why do they call it a 'waiting room'? It should really be called the 'waiting forever room'—where time stands still, and your anxiety levels rise!"

Cancer is no laughing matter, but finding humor in the journey can create moments of connection, lighten the emotional load, and remind us that even in the face of adversity, laughter can still coexist.

PAUSE FOR THOUGHT

Establishing a routine provides structure and stability, helping to create a sense of normalcy during uncertain times. However, making flexibility part of that routine allows us to adapt to the unpredictable nature of our illness, ensuring that we can respond to our needs and energy levels. Surrounding ourselves with moments of laughter, whether through light-hearted conversations or enjoyable activities, also plays a significant role in our overall health. Embracing joy in daily life not only uplifts our spirits but also provides emotional healing.

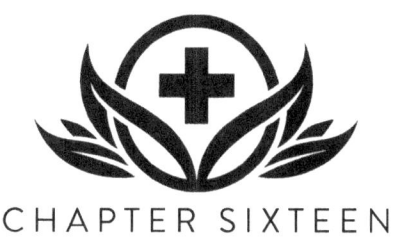

CHAPTER SIXTEEN

Rediscovering a Hobby

While living in the Philadelphia area, I found enjoyment and inspiration in capturing the historic buildings, churches, and unique locations with my camera. Each photograph was more than just an image; it was a story waiting to be told. I carefully organized these pictures, pairing them with commentary that reflected not only the beauty of the architecture but also the emotions and memories tied to each place.

As I faced the challenges of my illness, I returned to photography as a comforting hobby. It allowed me to reconnect with the world. Each photo captured not just visual beauty but also life itself, providing me with a therapeutic outlet. My renewed interest in photography helped me turn my thoughts and emotions into something meaningful, celebrating the moments that deserved to be remembered.

With my camera, I shifted my focus from historic buildings to the people and places around me, especially since I wasn't getting out as much. This rediscovered hobby became a way to express my emotions and find beauty in my surroundings.

Photography gave me a sense of purpose and connected me to the world around me. It encouraged me to notice the details often overlooked. I took photos of natural landscapes, such as the intricate details of blooming flowers and the unique shapes and colors of cacti, finding comfort in the calming presence of the outdoors. These images served as reminders of the beauty that exists beyond my illness, offering a sense of peace and connection to the world around me.

I also wanted to capture meaningful moments with family and friends, catching candid interactions and smiles that highlight the importance of relationships during this time. I loved taking pictures of my grandchildren, even when they often shied away from the camera, and documenting personal milestones and everyday routines.

Sharing my photographs has created connections and inspired others to see the world through my eyes. Each image tells a story, sparking emotions and conversations. Have you ever found that a distraction can help lighten the burden of your worries? What could you use as a distraction?

There are more positives in my life that I want to mention here. My love for reading is returning, and friends are supplying me with a good lending library. Social activities, previously limited to short visits, now include enjoyable outings like going to a friend's house for an evening barbecue or a morning meal.

My next-door neighbor remembered my love for breakfast and invited me over for pancakes and sausage. Another friend suggested lunch at a new restaurant known for its lobster rolls. I realized that these times together were easy to handle and truly brightened my day! Additionally,

I've started exploring other activities, which has brought a fresh sense of excitement to each day.

As I began to re-engage with the world around me, I discovered that these small outings were not just about the food or the company; they became important moments of connection. Sharing laughter over breakfast or reminiscing during lunch helped lift the weight of my illness, even if just for a little while. Each shared meal felt like a celebration of life, reminding me of the enjoyment that still existed amid the challenges I faced.

These small excursions also sparked conversations about future plans and dreams, reigniting a sense of hope and possibility within me. I understood that while the road ahead may be uncertain, the love and companionship of those around me can provide the strength I need to keep moving forward. I found myself dreaming aloud about places I wanted to visit and experiences I longed to have.

PAUSE FOR THOUGHT

Engaging in a hobby can serve as a wonderful distraction, providing a much-needed escape from the stresses of daily life. It allows us to immerse ourselves in something enjoyable, encouraging creativity and relaxation while also offering a sense of accomplishment and fulfillment. A hobby can also improve our mental health and create a sense of normalcy. By dedicating time to activities that bring us pleasure, we enhance our overall well-being and cultivate a positive outlook.

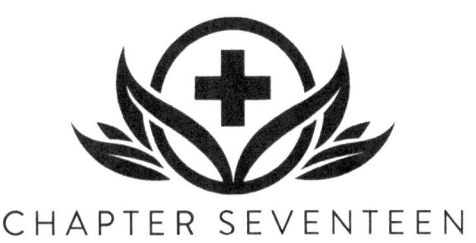

CHAPTER SEVENTEEN

Reflective Thoughts

I have been driving more and enjoying this new sense of freedom. There is no reason I should not be able to get out and take advantage of my independence. Since I am not taking any medications that affect my ability to drive, my confidence behind the wheel has grown.

Each time I get in the car, I feel as if I am regaining a part of my life that had been sidelined for too long. This freedom allows me to enjoy some spontaneity, which I have missed since my life became more scheduled.

During this time, I have also been trying to stretch my limits more, and while I have experienced some restless nights afterward, I see those as part of the journey. I have moved past the self-consciousness I once felt; I realize others may recognize my battle with cancer, but I no longer feel the need to draw attention to it. Instead, I find a sense of satisfaction in simply being myself, embracing moments of normalcy with those around me.

I must take a moment to share something that has captivated my attention: the development of a rose in my garden. While it has yet to bloom,

I can sense the promise it holds of becoming something incredibly beautiful. This rose symbolizes the growth of love in my life. Though I do not consider myself traditionally religious, my deeply religious upbringing still influences me. I remember the saying, "God is love," which has taken on a new meaning during this time in my life.

As I navigate this challenging period, I am increasingly aware of the amazing power of love—both in how it is expressed and its presence. Knowing that I am surrounded by loved ones is a source of comfort, reminding me of the essential human need to love and be loved. This realization has become clearer, much like the rose that is steadily growing in my garden.

I am committed to nurturing this blossoming understanding of love. I recognize that, like the rose, it requires patience and care to fully grow. Love is not something that simply happens; it needs to be cultivated through meaningful connections, shared experiences, and open communication. With dedication, I hope to fully embrace this love, enriching my life and the lives of those around me.

The love I have received from friends, family, and especially my wife has become a lifeline as I navigate the stress and uncertainty of my fight with cancer. There were moments when I felt as if I were fighting this battle alone, but the unwavering support and encouragement I have received have allowed me to continue taking positive steps forward.

Thinking about love reminds me of my worth and how important connections are in my life. It has lifted my spirits and provided comfort through the difficulties of my journey. Even seemingly small gestures, like my wife kissing me goodbye whenever she leaves, even for a brief time, take on profound significance. Each kiss becomes a reminder of her love and support, reinforcing my sense of connection and reminding me I am never truly alone.

Beyond personal achievements, the small gestures of beauty in my life have also made a significant difference. Every week, my wife brings home fresh flowers, a simple yet powerful reminder of beauty even during tough times. These flowers symbolize hope and renewal, creating a warm and inviting atmosphere that uplifts my spirits. Sharing stories, challenges, and triumphs with others who understand the impact of cancer has also provided a comforting perspective.

Together, these connections have created a holistic approach to my well-being, blending physical, emotional, and social aspects to help me navigate this challenging path with greater strength and optimism.

Off the subject, but important nonetheless, is whether there are activities that might be considered "off limits" for someone with a serious cancer diagnosis. For many, the desire to make the most of each moment can lead to a more adventurous spirit, helping them reevaluate what they want to do.

For instance, when my friend suggested playing a few holes of golf, I was initially unsure if I could handle it. But when I tried it, it turned out to be a very pleasant experience that lifted my spirits. These activities reminded me of the joy of being outdoors and connecting with friends, reinforcing the idea that life can still be enjoyed, even with serious health concerns.

I asked my doctor about his thoughts on the subject, and he reassured me that the benefits of pushing my boundaries far outweighed the challenges.

PAUSE FOR THOUGHT

Love can be a powerful source of strength and comfort during a cancer journey, providing emotional support and a sense of belonging. It encourages resilience as partners, family, and friends come together to navigate the challenges, reminding us of the importance of connection and compassion in the face of adversity. Love serves as a sign of hope, lighting the path ahead even in the darkest times. This unwavering support not only helps us endure difficult moments but also inspires us to treasure every shared experience along the way.

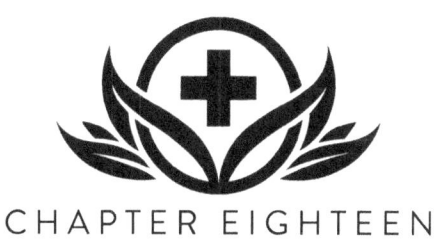

CHAPTER EIGHTEEN

Positive Days

I am feeling well and proud of my progress. It is like climbing a mountain—each step up feels like a win as I make my way to the top. I believe that the positive outlook I have developed will improve my quality of life moving forward.

Although my oncologist has mentioned that chemotherapy could improve my quality of life, it would likely come with significant side effects. Since my current treatment has been effective, he has chosen to delay suggesting it, having postponed its start three times now.

I am happy to hear that our son will be visiting this weekend with his family. Although my daughter's children are still too young to grasp the severity of my situation, I can sense that my son's kids understand a little more.

We spent time on our patio admiring my wife's gardening—a space filled with flowers that were in full bloom—and enjoyed a pleasant day. Our son has been visiting often, and I always look forward to our time together, enjoying the moments when we can simply be with each other without the weight of unspoken worries.

It is one thing to talk about my cancer with friends and relatives, but discussing my illness with my own children is tough and can feel awkward. It is a delicate balance, trying to share my reality while also protecting them from too much pain.

Our son and I have been able to talk about the subject in some detail, while our daughter gets too upset when I begin the conversation, often expressing her feelings through tears and withdrawing from the discussion altogether. Sometimes, just sitting together in silence can speak volumes. Since our daughter will be here next week for a few days, maybe we will have the opportunity to talk more openly.

I am also looking forward to her arrival with her two younger children, who did not come on the prior trip. The thought of their laughter filling the house is something I have missed. I'm excited about her visit because I feel so much better than I did during her last trip right after my diagnosis; it is amazing how much perspective a little time can provide.

I even feel well enough to go to the airport to meet them! It's a small outing, but it feels monumental to me. I have thought of some enjoyable activities we could do together— spending an afternoon at the beach, going to a local playground, and taking a few side trips I hope they will enjoy. These plans give me a sense of purpose and excitement as I prepare for their arrival.

There was also some significance to my daughter's visit. Earlier, I spoke of the feeling that my little world seemed to have stopped. There was no longer any need to plan ahead, for I could not know how I might feel. I was at least partly wrong. Three months ago, my daughter announced her intention of returning to see me.

I marked that in my mental calendar and felt confident that I would be up for the visit. I wanted to be as fit mentally and physically as possible. And so, I was. We had a wonderful visit. A simple insight, but significant, is that the world, my world, had not stopped. I have not stopped living! I must continue to think about how these days will be spent. I can and will set up short- term goals.

A cancer diagnosis can profoundly affect family and friends, often starting a complex emotional experience marked by grief, fear, and uncertainty. It is a journey that no one wants to take, yet it's one that many of us will face in some form.

Friends and family may experience a range of emotions, from shock and denial to anger and profound sadness, as they deal with the reality of possibly losing someone they care about. The diagnosis can disrupt family dynamics, forcing individuals to confront their own vulnerabilities and the impending loss.

When friends learned about my diagnosis, their support was everything I could have hoped for. Many checked in regularly to see how I was feeling and provided a listening ear, offering comfort and understanding when I needed it most. Their genuine concern made me feel less isolated in my struggle, reminding me that I was not alone in this fight.

Additionally, a few friends planned activities or outings to distract me from my concerns, whether it was going to a movie, taking a walk, or simply hanging out at home. These moments of normalcy became important in lifting my spirits and reminding me of the happy experiences that still existed in my life.

The effort they made to include me in their lives and create a sense of connection was a powerful reminder that friendship can be a source of healing. Simply being present, whether through calls, visits, or shared activities, made a significant difference in how I felt during this trying time.

Knowing I had a solid support system allowed me to lean into my feelings and navigate my journey with greater courage, reinforcing the idea that love and friendship are essential components of healing. It is a reminder that even during this struggle, there is still so much to treasure.

PAUSE FOR THOUGHT

As we navigate the complexities of illness and relationships, it is essential to remember that every moment spent with loved ones is a special gift that strengthens our connections. Embracing both the joy and the challenges of these experiences can deepen our appreciation for life and the relationships that matter most. These shared moments create lasting memories that keep us going through trying times. Ultimately, they remind us of the power of love and the importance of treasuring each day together.

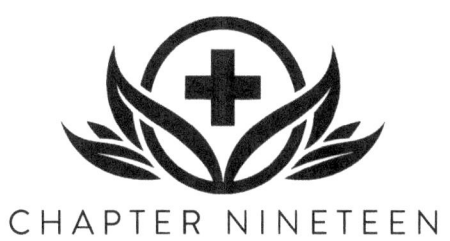

CHAPTER NINETEEN

Importance of Gratitude

I have started keeping notes and lists, which give me a certain satisfaction in organizing my thoughts and ideas. Writing down short-term goals brings a renewed sense of purpose and connection during this time. It is important for me to take a moment to express my gratitude to the people who continue to support me each day.

Life can get busy, and sometimes I may forget to appreciate the little things that make a difference. When someone takes the time to reach out, whether it's a simple note or an enjoyable chat over coffee, it brightens my day and reminds me I am not alone.

Gratitude has become a key part of my life as a cancer patient. It might sound surprising, given some issues I have faced. But when I take a moment to think about the good things in my life, it helps shift my mind away from fear and anxiety.

When I focus on the people, moments, and experiences I am grateful for, it provides me with a perspective that helps me cope. A simple "thank you" goes a long way in strengthening my connections with others, and it can make this journey feel a little less lonely.

Interestingly, I have found that practicing gratitude also positively affects my physical health. I am better about taking care of myself, whether that means sticking to my treatment plan, getting enough rest, or even enjoying a walk outside. It is as if recognizing what I am grateful for gives me the energy and motivation to prioritize my health, which is so important during this time.

Gratitude has boosted my happiness. Instead of getting lost in the fear and worry that cancer brings, I try to focus on what brings me enjoyment. One thing I have noticed is that gratitude inspires me to pay it forward. When I stop to think about the kindness I have received, it motivates me to extend that same compassion to others, whether it's offering a listening ear to someone else going through a tough time or simply sharing a smile.

One question that I have asked myself is, "Am I happy?" Reflecting on happiness with a serious cancer diagnosis brings a unique perspective. For many, the journey through illness can feel overwhelming, often overshadowing moments of enjoyment. However, this experience can also highlight what truly matters in life — my values, dreams, and the impact I hope to have on others, prompting me to rethink happiness itself.

The friendships I have built, especially the years spent golfing with the same group of guys, along with our friends and neighbors, are blessings I treasure. The laughter, camaraderie, and shared stories continue to enrich my life. And then there are my children and grandchildren. Watching them grow and develop has been a constant source of joy.

These gifts of family, friendship, and experiences, both big and small, shape who I am, and no illness can take away the gratitude I feel for all that I have had and continue to enjoy. Reflecting on my journey helps me appreciate each chapter that has brought its own lessons and adventures, shaping me into the person I am today.

On another note, every little symptom makes me think my cancer might be progressing. I realize this is a natural response to the uncertainty that comes with advanced cancer. I keep a close eye on my health to stay informed and address any issues quickly. This awareness can sometimes lead to anxiety, as I worry about what those symptoms might mean and how they could affect my treatment and quality of life.

I find myself stuck in a cycle of overthinking and self-diagnosing, which can be unsettling. However, I also know that not every change means my cancer is getting worse, and this helps ground me during uncertain times.

It is important to find a balance between staying aware of my health and keeping a sense of normalcy in my life. I have learned that engaging in everyday activities and focusing on the things I enjoy can help ease some of that anxiety. Staying connected with friends and family, pursuing hobbies, and even practicing mindfulness have become essential tools in managing my mental health.

I plan to speak openly with my doctors about any concerns I have so they can provide the support and guidance I need. Their insights reassure me and help relieve my fears, allowing me to focus more on living fully rather than being consumed by worry. By finding this balance, I can live in the moment while also planning for a healthy future.

I continue to read and find it a great distraction, and I enjoy listening to Pandres baseball games on the radio. Friends stop by for visits and often bring cookies or another treat because they know I have always had a sweet tooth—and I still do! What are you doing to take care of your mental health?

PAUSE FOR THOUGHT

Practicing gratitude during a cancer journey can provide a powerful perspective shift, allowing us to focus on the support of loved ones and the strength we must have to face challenges. By recognizing and appreciating even the small successes and moments of joy, we can develop a sense of hope and perseverance that sustains us throughout treatment and recovery. This positive mindset not only enriches our daily experiences but also helps us to approach each day with renewed energy and determination.

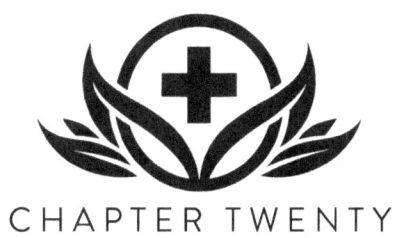

CHAPTER TWENTY

Changing Seasons

As October arrives, I am enjoying the colorful changes around me. The nights are getting cooler, while the days are still warm, creating a contrast that reminds me of the seasons of life. This shift feels significant as I navigate my illness and the changes it brings. As trees shed their leaves, it serves as a reminder that letting go can be a natural part of life. This process encourages me to reflect on what no longer holds meaning in my life, making space for new beginnings.

Each day presents new opportunities for growth, and I am learning to appreciate the small successes along the way. Each small step counts, and I must recognize it for the progress it is. The love from family and friends, along with the beauty of nature, inspires hope and reminds me that even in difficult times, there is always a reason to feel optimistic. I have a support system that lifts me up, especially when I need it the most.

Just as nature changes, I am experiencing my own renewal. Each day feels more valuable, and I find comfort in the simple pleasures of the season. Observing the changes around me motivates me to treasure each moment as I navigate this new chapter of my life. I have learned to tap into my inner resilience, especially on particularly hard days.

I remind myself to embrace each day, where every moment becomes an opportunity to create lasting memories. I love spending time with family and friends, whether it's sharing a cup of cider or enjoying gatherings filled with laughter and fun.

This journey is about resilience and hope, reminding me to appreciate this time as a gift. Halloween will soon be here, followed by Thanksgiving, one of my favorite holidays. It prompts me to think about the achievements I've made, the lessons learned, and the changes I have undergone. Thanksgiving provides a time for connection, allowing us to share stories, support one another, and reflect together on the gratitude we have for the experiences that have shaped us.

Reflecting on my experience with cancer, I am reminded that life is about the connections we create and the love we share. It's about celebrating the little things—a good laugh, a kind gesture, or a simple moment of understanding. My journey has strengthened my resolve to be a source of positivity and support for others, reinforcing the idea that even in tough times, we can find joy in our relationships and shared experiences.

I find happiness in reflecting on the positive influence I can continue to have on those around me. I do not want others to think of me solely as someone who battled cancer but, more importantly, as a loving partner, supportive friend, and caring family member. I want to encourage others to embrace their cancer journeys with courage and authenticity, creating a ripple effect of compassion and strength that resonates far beyond our time.

PAUSE FOR THOUGHT

Shifting seasons symbolize the natural cycle of life, reminding us that change, and renewal are part of our journey. Each season brings its own beauty and challenges, encouraging us to embrace this time, adapt to new circumstances, and find enjoyment in the distinct phases of our lives. Just as nature changes, we too can grow and develop in response to the experiences we face. This progression reminds us that even during difficulty, there is always the potential for renewal and new beginnings.

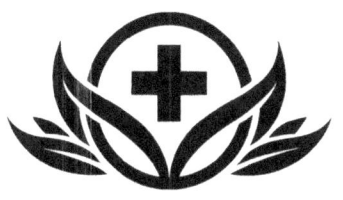

Epilogue

Going through a journey with cancer or any serious illness can profoundly alter your outlook on life. It is unfortunate that we sometimes need to go through an experience like this to appreciate how we should try to live each day. These are the lessons I have learned:

Cancer can teach the importance of living in the moment. Each day becomes a precious opportunity to experience life fully, leading to a greater appreciation of small joys and simple pleasures.

This journey encourages us to focus on what truly matters—spending time with family and friends. This often leads to deeper relationships and greater empathy for one another.

Understanding the value of self-care by prioritizing our health, mental well-being, and finding outlets for stress relief is important for each of us.

Developing a greater sense of gratitude for our lives and experiences helps us realize how valuable each moment can be, regardless of its nature.

Being true to ourselves, pursuing our interests, and living our lives according to our values, rather than conforming to others' expectations, is necessary for true happiness.

Looking for a deeper meaning and purpose in life helps us reflect on our goals and what truly matters.

By making these lessons part of our daily lives, I believe we will develop a deeper understanding, encourage growth, and ensure lasting positive change.

And you may ask, "Is that all?" And I would answer, "Yes, I believe it is."

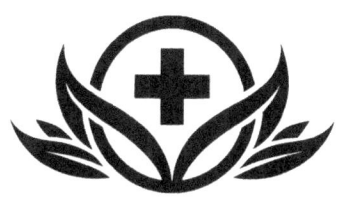

About the Authors

Arthur Moyer: I have always considered myself a fairly private person. I enjoyed a successful career in business, had a solid marriage, and led a fulfilling life. In my youth, I dreamed of becoming a writer, and throughout my life, I have approached challenges by examining them through the written word. So, when faced with the reality of my impending illness, it felt natural to document the experience as objectively as possible—almost like a journalist, which had been a long-held aspiration of mine.

My wife and I decided to move to California after living most of our lives in the Philadelphia area. I had just recently retired from my position at a large insurance company, and the allure of nice weather was very appealing. We could play golf and garden year-round, which were two of our favorite activities. We bought a home in Rancho Bernardo, just outside of San Diego, right on the golf course. We enjoyed getting to know our new location and meeting all the people in our neighborhood and surrounding community. Life was good!

Susie Watts: While cleaning out my desk drawers one day, I stumbled upon a long-forgotten manuscript buried beneath a collection of papers and miscellaneous items. Intrigued, I decided to pull it out and take a look. To my surprise, it was my father's story of his battle with cancer. As I skimmed through the pages, I was moved by his heartfelt writing, prompting me to read it more closely and reflect on his experience.
I knew it would require a considerable amount of rewriting, but I felt that I was up to the task.

My father and I were close, which made me hesitant to work on this writing project years ago, despite his encouragement for me to do so. I was also juggling four children under the age of nine, which kept me incredibly busy while managing a part-time job at my shop. Initially, I believed I could not do it; the thought of delving into those memories was not something I was ready to face. However, after many years of reflection and conversation with others, I decided to reconsider.

My children enjoyed many wonderful times with my father, and I was always sorry that they did not have more time with him as they grew older. I find great meaning in the lessons my father passed on and the love we shared. Revisiting these memories has proven to be a cathartic experience, allowing me to remember and celebrate his life. May our thoughts and reflections offer meaningful insights for your own journey.

I hope that this book brings comfort to those facing similar challenges. If you found it helpful, I would be truly grateful if you could share it with others who might benefit from its message. I also encourage you to leave a review on Amazon to help spread the word. Thank you for your support.